Anxious Art

Layout & Cover Design: Elina Diaz

For special orders, quantity sales, course adoptions and corporate sales, please email the publisher at sales@mango.bz. For trade and wholesale sales, please contact Ingram Publisher Services at customer.service@ingramcontent.com or +1.800.509.4887.

This book is not intended as an alternative or replacement to the medical advice of the reader's physicians. The reader should consult their doctor in all matters relating to their health prior to adjusting their diet.

Anxious Art: A Creativity Journal to Help Calm You

Library of Congress Cataloging-in-Publication number: 2019938545
ISBN: (print) 978-1-64250-100-1, (ebook) 978-1-64250-101-8
BISAC category code: GAM021000GAMES & ACTIVITIES / Guided Journals

Printed in the United States of America

Anxious Art

A Creativity Journal to Help Calm You

Yaddyra Peralta and Elina Diaz

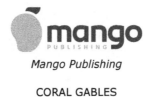

Mango Publishing

CORAL GABLES

inhale.

Table of Contents

Introduction

Poet T.S. Eliot famously said, "Anxiety is the handmaiden of creativity." But can anxiety somehow fuel the creative spirit of artmaking? Does that mean that artists must suffer to succeed? Not quite! What if you took Eliot's notion and tweaked it? What if creativity or creative activities could be used as a way to soothe anxiety?

Consider the results of a recent study published by Drexel art therapy professor, Girijai Kaimal, and her colleagues: whether you are a beginning or expert artist, creative activity reduces levels of cortisol, also known as the "stress hormone." The result is clear: reduce the cortisol, reduce anxiety and worry.

Taking part in creative activities is akin to taking part in any other kind of mindfulness activity, including meditation. Since you are focused on the task at hand—such as writing or painting—as well as accessing your imagination, you are distracted from your feelings of distress and anxiety. You then take part in what visual artist Louis Bourgeois powerfully describes as a healing process: "Art is restoration: the idea is to repair the damages that are inflicted in life, to make something that is fragmented—which is what fear and anxiety do to a person—into something whole."

When used as self-expression, creativity can allow you to take part in what psychologists call "sublimation" or the transformation of negative or socially unacceptable impulses into socially acceptable or even beautiful creations. Actor and comedian Jim Carrey has been open about his experiences with anxiety and depression. In the past few years, he has turned to painting. In the short documentary, *I Needed Color*, he says of his creations, "You can tell my inner life by the darkness in some of them, and you can tell what I want from the brightness in some of them." By using his imagination, Carrey not only documents his negative feelings but has made contact with the hope within. This is the kind of growth and transformation we all have access to.

How to Use This Book

The activities in this book are here to help you find tools for stress management. Dip in and out of the sections, trying them out in whatever order you prefer. While the long-term aim is to learn how to use the techniques to relieve feelings of dread or apprehension, do not place pressure on yourself to achieve a particular goal. Affirm, write, and color for the sake of each activity. Be patient. If there is growth to be had, it may take time. As the Chinese proverb says, "Be not afraid of growing slowly, be only afraid of standing still."

Section 1

Lyrical Affirmations

Simply put, affirmations can help you build self-confidence and overcome fear. It might seem like a weird or silly thing to do, especially in the midst of turmoil; however, as physical exercise helps to strengthen muscles, the regular practice of quick affirmations helps to develop a positive outlook, which has been known to help lessen anxiety. Make it an everyday habit—as habitual as a morning cup of coffee or breakfast. Choose an affirmation in this section that addresses a weakness or general sense of negativity you might be feeling. Or make up your own that positively embodies the mental space you aspire to occupy. (Examples: I am calm; I am confident). Bring your affirmation back into your day if you feel the need to recall the peace and tranquility you have somehow left behind.

"I don't need your opinion.
I'm not waiting for your okay.
I'll never be perfect, but at
least now I'm brave."

—Alicia Keys

"Look to the past
and remember a smile,
and maybe tonight
I can breathe for a while."

—Blink-182

"If I fail, if I succeed,
at least I'll live as I believe."

—Whitney Houston

"Pretty, pretty please, don't you ever, ever feel
like you're less than, less than perfect."

—P!nk

"I woke up this morning.
Gotta smile when I say that
shit. I woke up this morning."

—Chance the Rapper

" 'Cause though the
truth may vary,
this ship will carry our bodies
safe to shore."

—Of Monsters and Men

"You don't have to
try so hard.

You don't have to bend until
you break.

You just have to get up, get
up, get up, get up.

You don't have to change a
single thing."

—Colbie Caillat

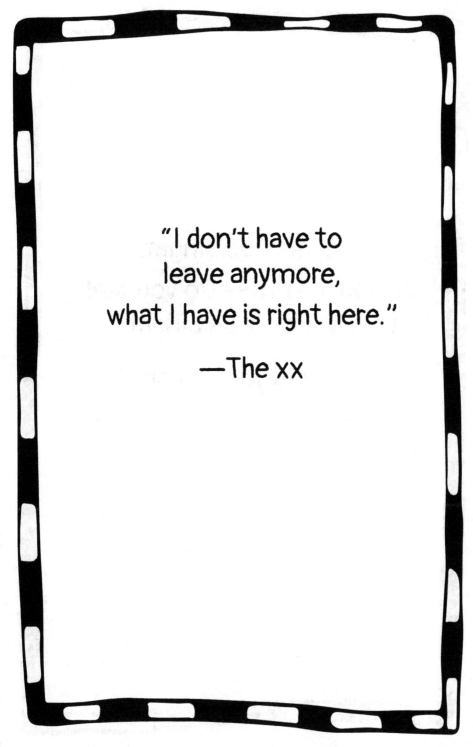

"I don't have to
leave anymore,
what I have is right here."

—The xx

"We gon' be alright.
Do you hear me? Do you feel
me? We gon' be alright."

—Kendrick Lamar

"They say it's happy here;
happiness is figurative.

I'm happy 'cause of me,
doesn't matter where
I'm living."

—The Neighbourhood

"I'm not the average
girl from your video
and I ain't built like
a supermodel,
but I learned to love
myself unconditionally
because I am a queen."

—India Arie

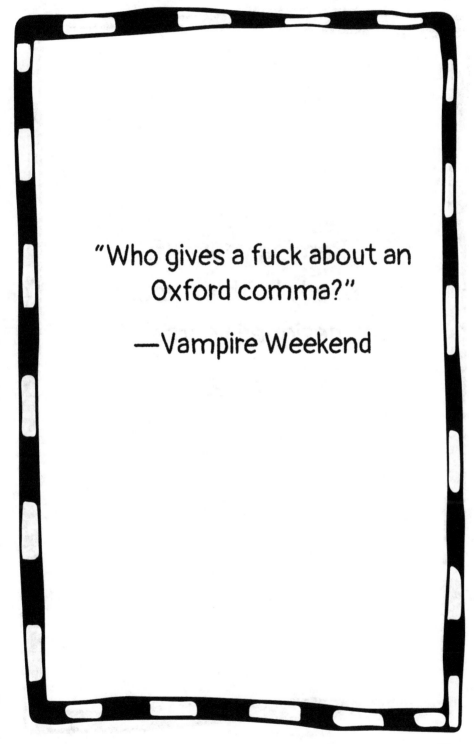

"Who gives a fuck about an Oxford comma?"

—Vampire Weekend

"Remind yourself:
nobody built like you.
You designed yourself."

—Jay-Z

"No need to give in,
there's nothing you
can't take,
'cause what you're made
of wasn't made to break.
You're even stronger,
stronger than you know.
You could stand together
or stand on your own."

—Jennifer Hudson

"I am recognizing that the voice inside my head is urging me to be myself but never follow someone else."

—A Tribe Called Quest

"Keep on dreamin', keep on believin', keep on achievin'.
I keep smiling when I come through, and I cry when I need to."

—Jill Scott

"Bad news comes, don't you worry even when it lands; good news will work its way to all them plans."

—Modest Mouse

"I'll put my armor on,
show you how strong I am."
—Sia

"Smile because you want to."

—Glass Animals

Section 2

Writer's Block(ing) Anxiety

Writing when you, the writer, are rooted in the present can be unbelievably cathartic and even joyful. It's not about impressing a teacher or a loved one. It's about staying grounded in what you are writing and focusing on the visualization of the ideas, memories, or imaginings that are helping your words to flow. It can be like talking to a therapist or even a best friend who understands your joys and fears and appreciates your sense of humor or outlook on the world.

Very Short Short Stories

Feel free to write a story that goes beyond the pages we provide here or a story that's a sentence long. Whatever gets your creative juices flowing.

_____

_____

_____

_____

_____

_____

_____

_____

_____

_____

_____

_____

_____

_____

_____

Write a short story about the first time you remember feeling anxious.

_____

_____

_____

_____

_____

_____

_____

_____

_____

_____

_____

_____

_____

_____

_____

_____

_____

_____

_____

_____

_____

_____

_____

_____

_____

_____

_____

_____

_____

_____

_____

_____

_____

_____

_____

_____

_____

_____

_____

_____

_____

_____

_____

_____

_____

_____

_____

Write a short story set on the moon.

_____

_____

_____

_____

_____

_____

_____

_____

_____

_____

_____

_____

_____

_____

_____

_____

_____

_____

_____

_____

_____

Write a short story about being stuck in the middle seat during an eight-hour flight.

_____

_____

_____

_____

_____

_____

_____

_____

_____

_____

_____

_____

_____

_____

_____

_____

_____

_____

Write a short story only using alliteration. (You can cheat a little.)

_____

_____

_____

_____

_____

_____

_____

_____

_____

_____

_____

_____

_____

_____

_____

_____

_____

_____

_____

_____

_____

_____

_____

_____

_____

_____

_____

_____

_____

_____

_____

_____

_____

_____

_____

_____

_____

_____

_____

_____

_____

_____

_____

_____

_____

_____

Write a short story about the calmest place you can imagine, real or fictional.

_____

_____

_____

_____

_____

_____

_____

_____

_____

_____

_____

_____

_____

_____

_____

_____

_____

_____

_____

Write a short story only using lyrics from an album.

_____

_____

_____

_____

_____

_____

_____

_____

_____

_____

_____

_____

_____

_____

_____

_____

_____

_____

_____

_____

_____

_____

_____

_____

_____

_____

_____

_____

_____

_____

_____

_____

_____

_____

_____

_____

_____

_____

_____

_____

_____

_____

_____

_____

_____

Write a short story about stopping for gas in Nebraska during a cross-country road trip.

_____

_____

_____

_____

_____

_____

_____

_____

_____

_____

_____

_____

_____

_____

_____

_____

_____

_____

_____

_____

_____

_____

_____

_____

_____

_____

_____

_____

_____

_____

_____

_____

_____

_____

_____

_____

_____

_____

_____

_____

_____

_____

_____

_____

Write a short story about writing short stories to cope with anxiety.

_____

_____

_____

_____

_____

_____

_____

_____

_____

_____

_____

_____

_____

_____

_____

_____

_____

_____

_____

_____

Write a short story inspired by the last dream you remember.

_____

_____

_____

_____

_____

_____

_____

_____

_____

_____

_____

_____

_____

_____

_____

_____

_____

_____

_____

_____

_____

Write a short story with no human characters.

_____

_____

_____

_____

_____

_____

_____

_____

_____

_____

_____

_____

_____

_____

_____

_____

_____

_____

Write a short story about the existential crisis of being the first human to discover that we are living in a video game simulation.

_____

_____

_____

_____

_____

_____

_____

_____

_____

_____

_____

_____

_____

_____

_____

_____

_____

_____

_____

Write a short story in which Chapstick plays a pivotal role.

_____

_____

_____

_____

_____

_____

_____

_____

_____

_____

_____

_____

_____

_____

_____

_____

_____

_____

_____

_____

_____

_____

_____

_____

Write a short story about sunflowers and vinyl records on a night stand.

_____

_____

_____

_____

_____

_____

_____

_____

_____

_____

_____

_____

_____

_____

_____

_____

_____

_____

Plays with Way-Too-Specific Rules

Write a play in which two characters argue over putting ketchup or mustard on hot dogs while waiting for a hot dog vendor who never shows up.

_____

_____

_____

_____

_____

_____

_____

_____

_____

_____

_____

_____

_____

_____

_____

_____

_____

_____

Write a play in which your anxiety is a character.

_____

_____

_____

_____

_____

_____

_____

_____

_____

_____

_____

_____

_____

_____

_____

_____

_____

_____

_____

_____

_____

_____

_____

_____

_____

_____

_____

_____

_____

_____

_____

_____

_____

_____

_____

_____

_____

_____

_____

_____

_____

_____

_____

_____

_____

_____

_____

_____

_____

_____

_____

_____

_____

_____

_____

_____

_____

_____

_____

_____

_____

_____

_____

_____

_____

Write a play about angels trying to cross the border into the US, only to encounter the devil.

_____

_____

_____

_____

_____

_____

_____

_____

_____

_____

_____

_____

_____

_____

_____

_____

_____

_____

Write a play that has exactly four characters (one of which is a potted plant).

_____

_____

_____

_____

_____

_____

_____

_____

_____

_____

_____

_____

_____

_____

_____

_____

_____

_____

_____

Write a play where dinosaurs are brought back to life as a stunt to create an amusement park; call it "Billy and the Cloneasaurous"... wait, never mind, that already exists. Instead, just try watching *Jurassic Park*.

_____

_____

_____

_____

_____

_____

_____

_____

_____

_____

_____

_____

_____

_____

_____

_____

_____

_____

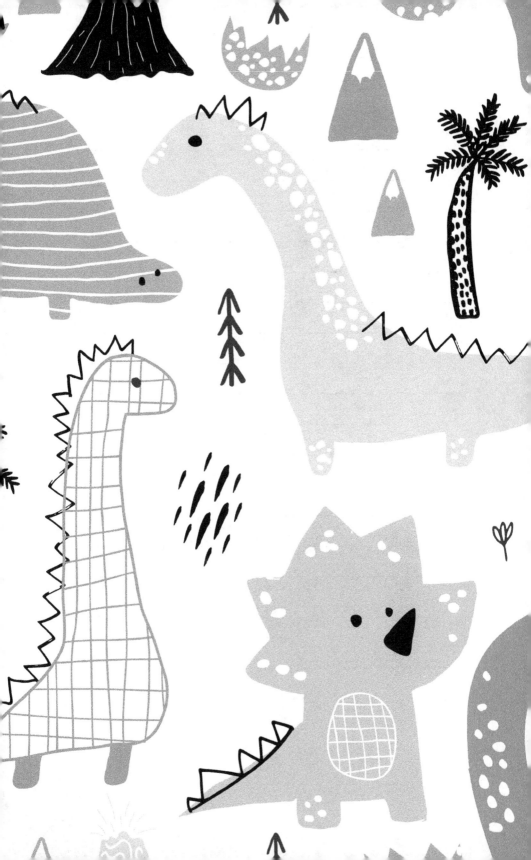

Write a monologue, single-act play about croissants from the perspective of a baker on their shop's opening day.

_____

_____

_____

_____

_____

_____

_____

_____

_____

_____

_____

_____

_____

_____

_____

_____

_____

Rewrite *Hamlet* using farm animals as characters.

_____

_____

_____

_____

_____

_____

_____

_____

_____

_____

_____

_____

_____

_____

_____

_____

_____

_____

_____

_____

Write a play that rhymes.

_____

_____

_____

_____

_____

_____

_____

_____

_____

_____

_____

_____

_____

_____

_____

_____

_____

_____

_____

_____

_____

_____

_____

_____

_____

_____

_____

_____

_____

_____

_____

_____

_____

_____

_____

_____

_____

_____

_____

_____

_____

_____

_____

The Never-Ending Stream of Consciousness Poem

Start a poem. When you're ready stop, just stop and don't read it. When you come back to it, pick up where you left off. That's the only rule. Well, that and it needs to be like this sentence and just ramble but also feel light and cautious like good poetry. Not assertive, except when you feel it calls to be assertive.

_____

_____

_____

_____

_____

_____

_____

_____

_____

_____

_____

_____

_____

_____

_____

_____

_____

_____

_____

_____

_____

_____

_____

_____

_____

_____

_____

_____

_____

_____

_____

_____

_____

_____

_____

_____

_____

_____

_____

_____

_____

_____

_____

_____

_____

_____

_____

_____

_____

_____

_____

_____

_____

_____

_____

_____

_____

_____

_____

_____

_____

_____

_____

_____

_____

_____

_____

_____

_____

_____

_____

_____

_____

_____

_____

_____

_____

_____

_____

_____

_____

Yup, keep going!

_____

_____

_____

_____

_____

_____

_____

_____

_____

_____

_____

_____

_____

_____

_____

_____

_____

Section 3

Sketch Book

Doodles, those squiggly designs you drew on the edge of your notebook paper during high school math, provide more than the obvious benefit of entertaining you when you're bored. They have been said to help improve visual and factual recall. And, if you go back to the math class scenario (or any like it), consider whether you were drawing patterns because you were bored or because you were uncomfortable. Doodling, especially in a repetitive way, can slow down a racing mind in moments of anxiety.

As with meditation or doodling, coloring is an engaging activity that can allow you to turn off the over-thinking part of your brain. A great benefit of this is the reduction of free-floating anxiety. Over time, tranquility can be a result of coloring as a habit.

The best thing about doodling, coloring, or drawing is the sense that there is no right or wrong way to do it. And the results, often not predetermined, can be a beautiful surprise.

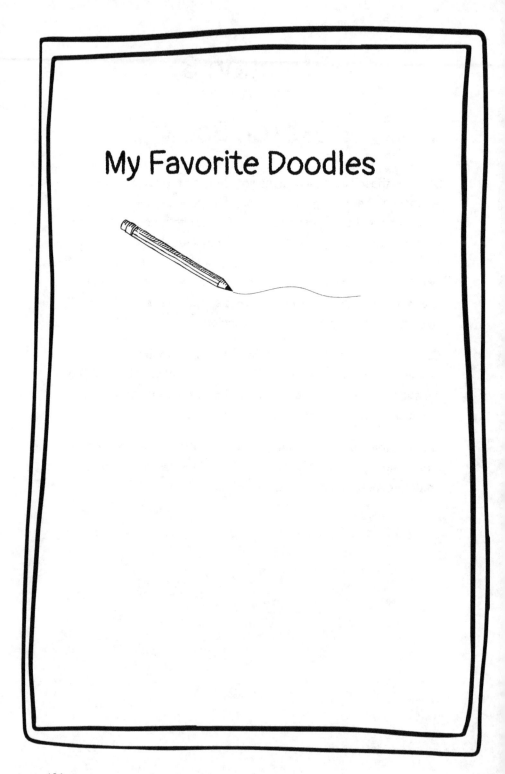

My Favorite Doodles

Doodle yourself.

Doodle your first crush.

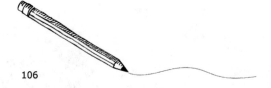

Doodle your latest crush.

Doodle your first crush fighting your latest crush.

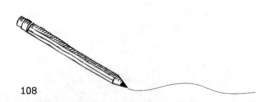

Doodle some of your favorite animals (or people).

Doodle your favorite number.

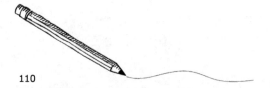

Doodle your least favorite number.

Doodle a lot of spirals.

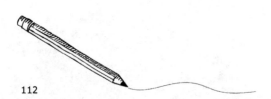

Doodle oodles of noodles.

Doodle things that rhyme with doodle like poodles and kudos (good luck).

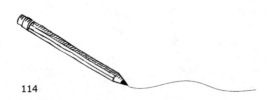

Doodle a scene from the hot dog play.

Doodle your biggest fear.

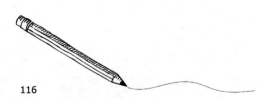

Doodle your biggest source of joy.

Doodle your self-portrait with your eyes closed.

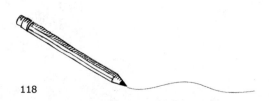

Doodle a sky full of stars.

Doodle what music sounds like.

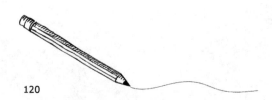

Doodle what your favorite food tastes like.

Doodle a snail going on a trip.

Doodle something that will make you cry.

Doodle something that will make you laugh.

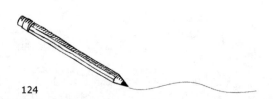

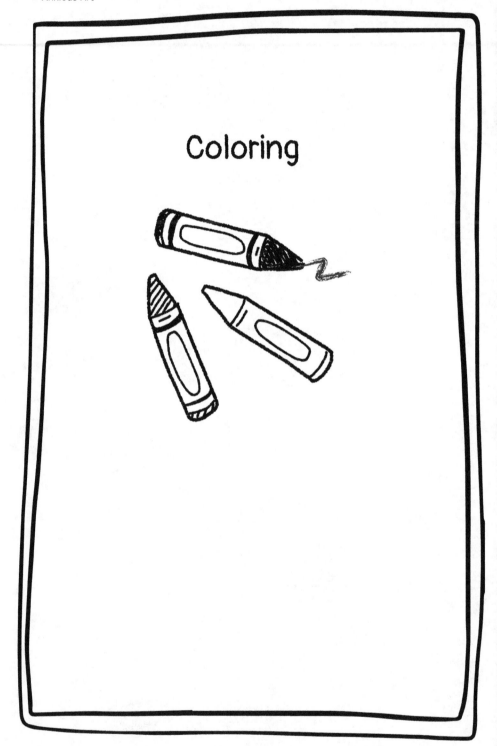

Coloring

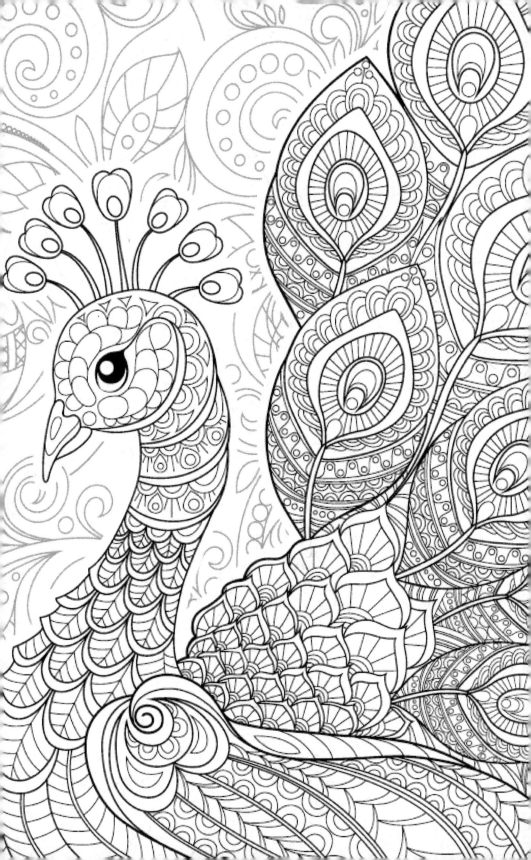

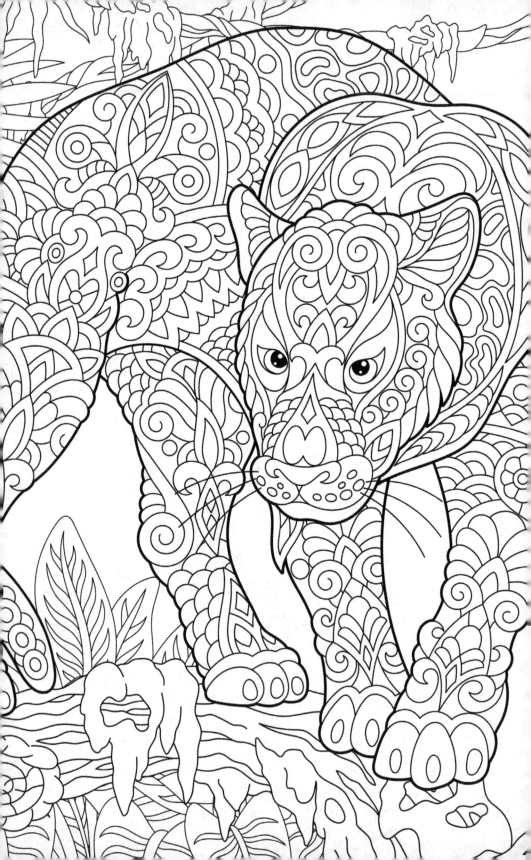

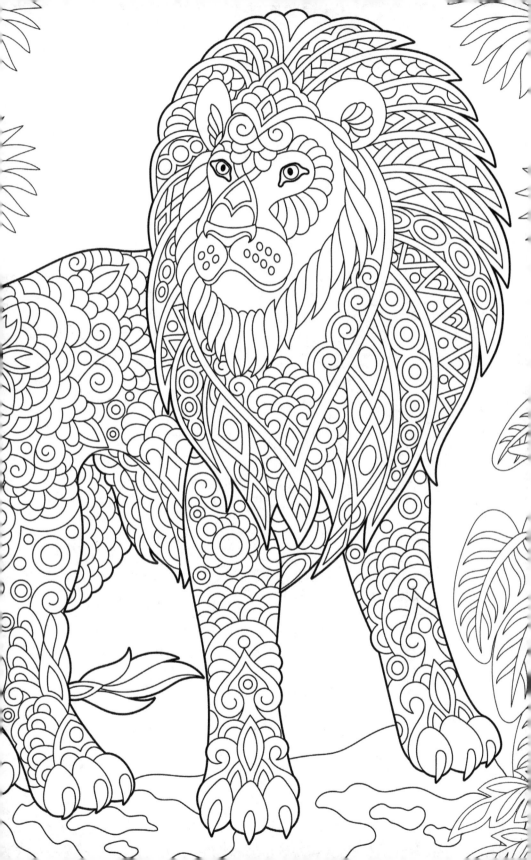

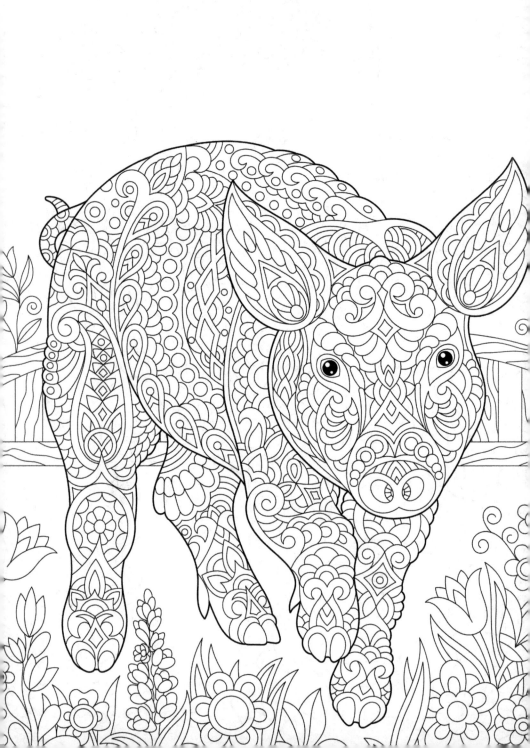

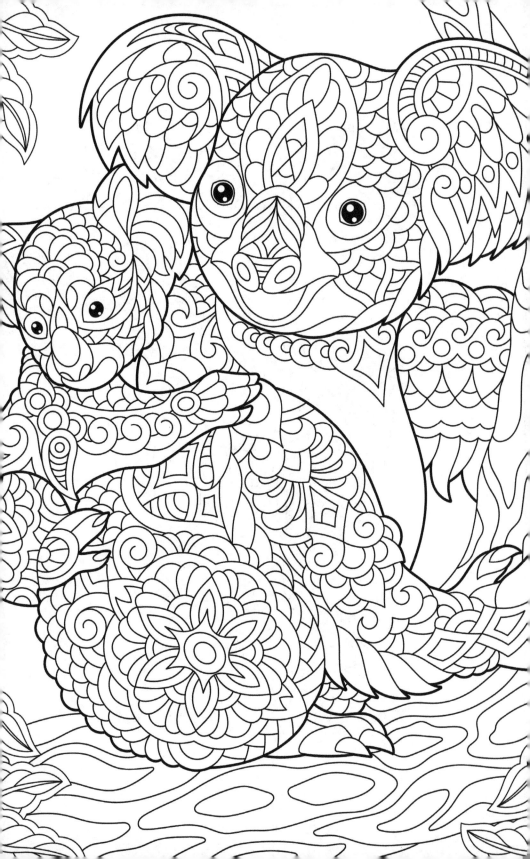

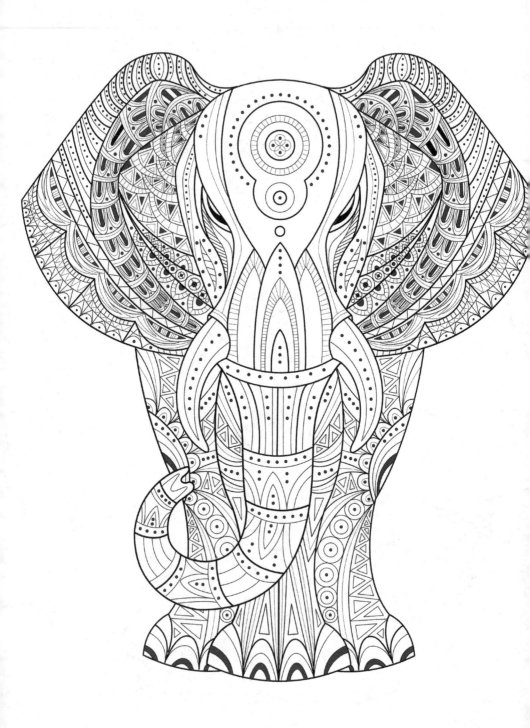

Rockin' Out

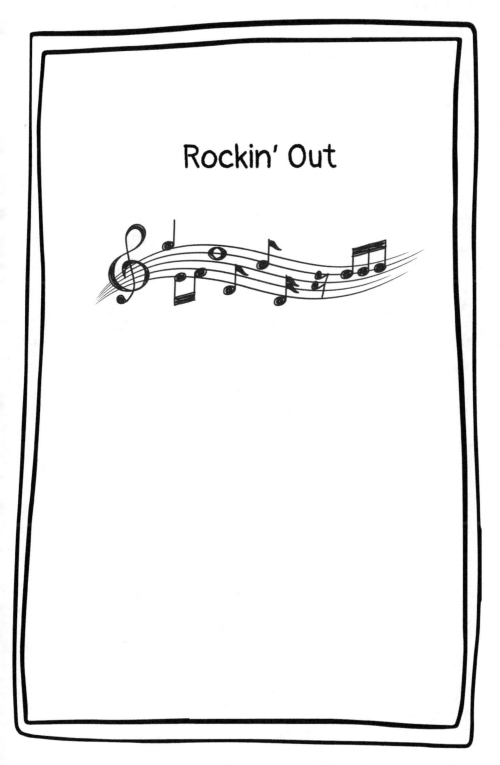

Name your make-believe band.

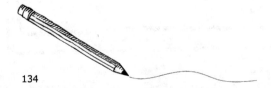

What genre of music do they play? Has it changed since they started? Doodle what the genre looks like.

Draw the band members.

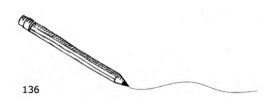

Give the band members names and bios.

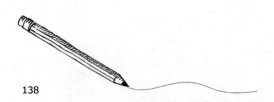

Title their first album (and their next three).

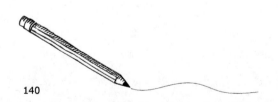

Draw some of their biggest fans.

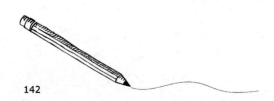

List some of their song titles.

Write some of their most liked tweets.

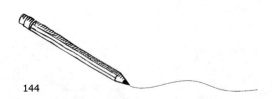

Sketch them some cover art.

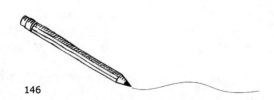

Section 4

Breathing Journal

There are a lot of misconceptions about mindfulness activities, particularly meditation. The idea is not just to empty your mind of thoughts, but to focus on the breath, an important constant of life. Turning away from distracting thoughts and back to the breath encourages you to realize that thoughts and feeling are often impermanent. A bad day is a bad day. It doesn't have to determine the rest of your week or year, especially if you choose to return to that which roots you, as a habit.

Meditation and other breathing exercises focus on the breath, but, more specifically, the lengthening of the intake and outtake of air, something that is often neglected, especially in dire times of stress. Slowing down to focus on breathing, like other activities mentioned in this book, brings you into the present moment, slows down your racing thoughts and heart rate, and reminds you to honor that which gives you life.

For this final section, simply start meditating. Try five minutes a day and gradually increase your time. After you are done meditating, journal down the thoughts, ideas, memories, and emotions that were flowing during your search for calm.

A Poem to End the Journey

Sanctuary

The world rushes in,
colliding with my feelings, like
speeding cars in
oncoming lanes.
I want to be an animal:
my eye made only to
gently follow
the simple changes in the air.
Words spun from my fingertips
fly through the air,
gently enveloping me
to make the kind of home
a snail carries on her back.

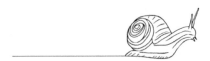

CPSIA information can be obtained
at www.ICGtesting.com
Printed in the USA
LVHW010833221220
674796LV00001B/1